SCHIZOPHRENIA EXPLAINED

Siegfried Kasper

Department of General Psychiatry
University of Vienna, Austria

ALTMAN

Published by Altman Publishing, 7 Ash Copse, Bricket Wood, St Albans, Herts, AL2 3YA, England

First edition 2003

Typeset in 10/12.5 Optima by Scribe Design, Gillingham, Kent
Printed in Great Britain by George Over Ltd, Rugby

ISBN 1 86036 023 8

A catalogue record for this book is available from the British Library

∞ Printed on acid-free text paper, manufactured in accordance with ANSI/NISO Z39.48-1992 (Permanence of Paper)

CONTENTS

ABOUT THE AUTHOR

Siegfried Kasper FRCPsych MD is Professor of Psychiatry and Chairman of the Department of General Psychiatry in the University of Vienna, Austria. He has worked both as a medical doctor and as a research scientist at hospitals in Austria, Germany and the United States. Dr Kasper has written over 800 scientific articles, mostly dealing with the biological basis of mental disorders and their treatment. He has also spoken on these topics at many national and international meetings. Currently, he is President of the Austrian Society of Neuropsychopharmacology and Biological Psychiatry.

PREFACE

Schizophrenia is a condition that is misunderstood by many people who do not regard it as a 'real' disease but rather a result of a disadvantaged upbringing or other social deprivation. This book not only serves to correct this mistaken impression, but also to provide information about the disease and its treatment. It will therefore be of real benefit both to sufferers and their families and to carers.

The author is a Professor of Psychiatry in the University of Vienna, Austria, so readers can be assured that the information contained in the book is up to date and medically and scientifically accurate. It is, of course, not meant to replace medical advice given by your own doctor but will serve to answer many more questions than your doctor is likely to have time for. It will be invaluable to patients and family members but will also be useful for health professionals who wish to know more about this condition.

1 INTRODUCTION

Schizophrenia is a complex disorder and not easy to define and study. However, substantial efforts have been made to uncover the biological, psychological and social origins of the condition, and the influence of these variables on the cause of the illness. The aim of this book is to summarize the existing knowledge on the disease on a very practical level, and it is hoped that this will be a useful guide for patients and carers. It is not possible to cover all the topics comprehensively but it is hoped that enough information is provided that is interesting and useful to the readership.

The condition known as *schizophrenia* is subdivided by doctors into a number of subgroups (see Table 6.1). These are given specific numbers in the World Health Organization's International Classification of Diseases. This is a complete catalogue of all known medical conditions and is now in its tenth edition. It is known, for short, as the ICD-10.

Schizophrenia research is currently advancing rapidly and this will lead to better treatments and understanding of the disorder. Many doctors believe that if a patient knows more about the disease, what causes it and what can be done about it, there will be better cooperation between patients, doctors, nurses and mental health specialists. This will help ensure that the best possible care is provided.

2 WHAT IS SCHIZOPHRENIA AND WHO GETS IT?

Schizophrenia affects about 1% of the population world wide, and this figure is more or less the same in all countries. Men and women are affected in equal numbers, although it seems that on average men develop it 2–3 years earlier than women.

The term schizophrenia probably means different things to different people, but most importantly, it has to be viewed as a *brain disease*. It is a disease like diabetes, epilepsy or high blood pressure, and like these diseases, there are numerous subtypes and variations. However, many people incorrectly think that schizophrenia is not a 'real' disease like, for example, diabetes, but is a personality disorder caused by, for

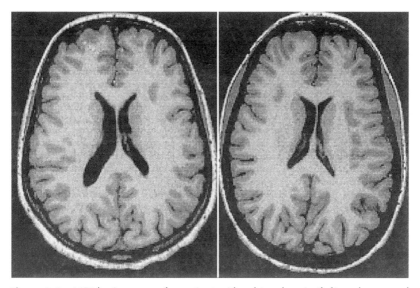

Figure 2.1 MRI brain scans of a patient with schizophrenia (left) and a normal scan (right) for comparison. The black areas (actually spaces) in the centre of the brain, called the ventricles, are larger in the patient with schizophrenia. (From *European Archives of Psychiatric and Clinical Neuroscience*, 1999, **249**, 4)

3

example, a troubled childhood, or a reaction to living in a complex and sometimes troubled world. Some of these ideas have found widespread acceptance in the press and other literature, but it is important to state that none of these theories is supported by scientific evidence.

There are actually some structural differences that can be seen on brain scans of some patients with schizophrenia. An example is shown in Figure 2.1.

There is also a great deal of scientific and medical evidence that in schizophrenia there is a disturbance in the transmission of nerve impulses within the brain due to a defect in the so-called dopaminergic

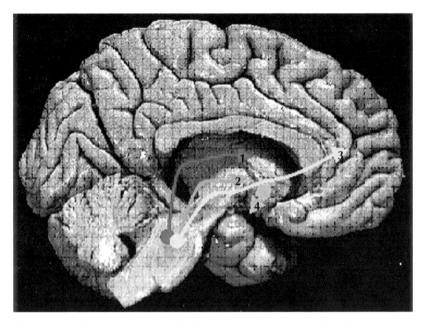

Figure 2.2 Diagram showing where dopamine pathways exist in the brain and the effects of either a high or low dopamine level. 1, Nigrostriatal pathway: dopamine OK. 2, Mesolimbic pathway: dopamine high. High dopamine leads to positive symptoms (hallucinations, delusions, emotional disturbance). 3, Mesocortical pathway: dopamine low. Low dopamine leads to negative symptoms (apathy, disturbed cognition, etc.). 4, Tuberoinfundibular pathway: dopamine OK.

system. This is a series of pathways where a chemical called dopamine is transmitted across parts of the brain. Figure 2.2 gives some more information on this topic.

Schizophrenia can also be thought of as a psychotic disorder. This means that the individual loses contact with external reality, in other words, his or her perceptions and interpretations of the world are different from those of other people. It is, of course, a difference of degree and is not an absolute statement. In schizophrenia there is usually a profound disorganization of mental functioning in the sense that external behaviour seems bizarre to observers and the patient is frightened by internal mental experiences.

Schizophrenia is not a split personality. The term schizophrenia was first used in 1911 by Professor Eugen Bleuler, a famous Swiss psychiatrist. Although the word does come from two Greek words meaning 'split' and 'mind', people with schizophrenia do not have split personalities, and it was not Professor Bleuler's intention to convey this idea. However, this misunderstanding has caused many people to misuse the term schizophrenia. The 'split mind' refers to the way that sufferers are split off from reality and when experiencing their symptoms cannot distinguish between what is real and what is not real.

It is important to understand that schizophrenia is a general term that encompasses a varied group of disorders. Just like people with diabetes or high blood pressure, patients with schizophrenia can differ in their precise symptoms, the severity of their condition, and their response to treatment. As is shown in Table 6.1, a number of specific subdivisions have been defined, and these are described in more detail in later pages.

The disability resulting from schizophrenia is high. The disease results in significant disadvantages that make a person unable to function on a par with others. However, the term disability should not mean that the person should be discriminated against. Moreover, the term should highlight that, like other disabled persons, the individual might function at nearly normal levels under the right circumstances, which involve environmental modifications and intensive rehabilitation programmes. The social consequences of schizophrenia can include isolation, ostracism, prejudice, mistreatment, unemployment, substandard housing, homelessness, poor education and lack of essential human services. Sometimes sufferers will be treated as criminals rather than as

5

sick people, or exploited in other ways by prolonged confinement without treatment. The health risks of schizophrenia can include an increased rate of other illnesses and early death, poor living conditions such as malnutrition and exposure to toxins, substance abuse, and suicide. However, on a positive note, newer and better antipsychotic drugs and rehabilitation programmes now exist so that much of the above is now no longer relevant.

3 WHAT ARE THE CAUSES OF SCHIZOPHRENIA?

With some diseases, the cause is well known. Diabetes, for example, is due to a lack of insulin. The situation is not quite so clear cut in the case of schizophrenia and it is likely that there is more than one cause. Although all of them are not yet known, there are several aspects that are known.

Genetics

Studies on twins have shown that there is definitely a genetic component to schizophrenia although it is not the only one. In sets of identical twins where one has schizophrenia, between 30 and 50% of the other twins will also have the illness. This means that genetics cannot be the only factor, otherwise all of the other twins would also have it.

Environment

The rate of schizophrenia found in the general population is about 1%. Studies on non-identical twins have found that where one has schizophrenia, the other twin will also have it in about 15% of cases. This is much more than in the general population, and points strongly to an environmental factor or factors as part of the cause. Such factors could include stress, poor social conditions, or an accident or infection at an early age. In some way, it seems that the genetic make-up of an individual comes together with their particular environment to cause schizophrenia.

4 WHAT ARE THE SYMPTOMS OF SCHIZOPHRENIA?

Doctors have classified the symptoms of schizophrenia into various main groups. These are:

- POSITIVE SYMPTOMS
- NEGATIVE SYMPTOMS
- AFFECTIVE SYMPTOMS
- COGNITIVE SYMPTOMS

Positive symptoms are hallucinations and delusions. *Hallucinations* can be defined as *unreal perceptions of one's surroundings.* These can include the following:

- hearing voices (auditory hallucinations)
- hearing commands to perform certain acts (command hallucinations)
- seeing things that are not there (visual hallucinations)
- experiencing unusual sensations of taste (gustatory hallucinations)
- inappropriate body movements (kinaesthetic hallucinations)
- feeling things that are not there (tactile hallucinations).

Auditory hallucinations are the most common ones in schizophrenia. Where this takes the form of a voice commanding the person to perform some action, sometimes a dangerous or violent one (command hallucination), the outcome can be serious if the patient acts upon the command.

If someone is experiencing any of the other types of hallucination (other than auditory ones), then it is highly likely that they are not suffering from schizophrenia but that some other mental disorder may be responsible. This obviously requires a detailed examination by a specialist.

Delusions can be defined as *bizarre and false beliefs.* These are usually of two basic types. Delusions of *paranoia* are those where the person has an unreal fear or suspicion that someone is 'out to get them'.

Delusions of *reference* are those where the person thinks the actions of other persons or neutral objects or events have a special meaning for the person. Delusions of *being controlled* means that the person's thoughts, feelings, impulses, or actions are controlled by aliens, spies, or other external forces rather than being under the personal control of the patient. Delusions of *grandeur* are those where the person believes that he or she is someone of great importance, such as the monarch or Prime Minister. (This symptom is often prominent in *bipolar disorder* – a condition where sufferers alternate between a manic state and a depressive state – and not in schizophrenia).

In rare situations, patients may also exhibit *catatonic behaviour* where they either become immobile and fixed in a single position, or where they experience severe agitation. However, it should be emphasized that these are quite rare manifestations of schizophrenia.

Negative symptoms means the *reduction or absence of normal behaviour*, that is, normal things, like interaction with friends, colleagues, or taking care of everyday belongings, are just happening to a lesser extent or don't happen at all. This is different from the positive symptoms of schizophrenia, hallucinations and delusions, which can be called the *presence of abnormal behaviour* (that is, abnormal things do happen). Negative symptoms therefore include a *lack of motion, social withdrawal, lack of expression, lack of energy and motivation*. A consequence of these feelings is that sometimes people with schizophrenia can lose interest in their personal hygiene.

Affective symptoms are mostly depressive symptoms or anxiety symptoms. These usually result in abnormalities of thinking and speech. People with schizophrenia often do not speak very much, or if they do, the speech can be disjointed and difficult to understand. The disorganized speech is quite characteristic for schizophrenia.

The negative and cognitive symptoms are those which cause the patient the largest problems in his or her social environment and are of the utmost importance for psychosocial rehabilitation programmes. An interest in relationships and interactions with other people and an ability to initiate and persist in goal-directed activities are essential components of everyday life. Many people with schizophrenia will lack at least some of these attributes, with the result that they find great difficulty in integrating into a normal social environment.

10

Cognitive symptoms are core symptoms of schizophrenia and imply difficulties in logical thinking, concentrating, developing plans and recognizing complex social situations. Most importantly, this means that in everyday living, the psychosocial environment is considered to be difficult to manage, and patients often withdraw and prefer to be alone.

5 THE IDEAL CONSULTATION: WHAT MY DOCTOR SHOULD KNOW

When the patient goes to see a doctor or another health care special-ist about the symptoms of schizophrenia, this should feel like a conver-sation between equals rather than an interrogation. It should be clear that the reason for going to see a doctor is to ensure that you receive the best possible treatment. The doctor has the responsibility to give enough time to explain all about the disease, to collect enough infor-mation to make an informed diagnosis, and to prescribe the most useful medication or initiate other treatments.

Of course it is most helpful if the patient can tell the doctor every-thing he or she may need to know so that the best help can be provided. In schizophrenia, due to the nature of the disorder, the patient does not necessarily view hallucinations or delusions as something abnormal. However, when the disease proceeds and when there is an under-standing with the doctor, both the patient and the doctor know that these hallucinations or delusions are symptoms of the disease. There is an insight into the illness, just like with diabetes when the patient realizes that the symptoms of hypoglycaemia (low blood sugar levels) are an expression of the disease. If the doctor uses any words that the patient does not understand, he or she should ask to have these explained. The patient should take as much time as is needed. This is a worthwhile use of time and the patient should never have the feeling that the doctor's time is being wasted.

Before a visit to see the doctor, and afterwards as well, it is useful to write down some questions, because just like in other situations when one is nervous, one tends to forget. It would be very frustrating to remember an important question when the consultation is over and the patient is back home.

The doctor or nurse will probably ask some of the following questions, and it would be useful to have a separate note of these before the consultation so that some thought can be given to the answers beforehand.

- How do you feel lately?
- Do you meet friends just as you did when you were well?
- Do you take your medication?
- Do you take your medication regularly?
- Do you have any trouble sleeping?
- Are you tense and anxious?
- Do you have symptoms of depression? Are you *down?*
- Have you lost your appetite? Have you lost weight?
- Do you have any feelings of aggression or hostility?
- Has anyone told you that you do things that other people do not understand?
- Do you have the feeling that other people laugh about you or that they speak about you?
- Has any member of your family or your friends told you that you have behaved strangely?
- Do you have difficulty in concentrating?

The patient should have a note of the following:

- the symptoms that he or she thinks are the most troublesome;
- when these symptoms started;
- when the patient feels best;
- when the patient feels worst;
- family history of any psychiatric diseases;
- any other diseases that the patient has had;
- all medicines currently taken by the patient;
- which medication in the past was good and which was not good;
- what kind of non-psychiatric medication the patient takes right now.

Armed with the above information, the doctor will be able to take into account the patient's full medical history as well as his or her own thoughts and feelings. In this way, it is much more likely that the patient will receive the best advice and the best care as regards future treatment.

6 HOW IS SCHIZOPHRENIA DIAGNOSED?

According to ICD-10, the diagnosis of schizophrenia is established on existing symptoms (as well as the exclusion of an organic illness, such as a brain tumour or encephalitis, for example), and furthermore that these symptoms have been present for a certain period of time. A diagnosis of schizophrenia, according to ICD-10, is *only given if a patient has delusions or auditory hallucinations for at least one month, or if there is disorganization of speech associated with negative symptoms also for at least one month.*

There are different subgroups of schizophrenia which are dependent on the symptoms. These are outlined in Table 6.1.

Table 6.1 The diagnostic categories of schizophrenia and their main symptoms according to ICD-10

F20.0	Paranoid schizophrenia: strong delusions or hallucinations
F20.1	Disorganized (hebephrenic) schizophrenia: lack of emotion; disorganized speech
F20.2	Catatonic schizophrenia: reduced or exaggerated movement, rigid posture
F20.3	Undifferentiated schizophrenia: mainly negative symptoms
F20.6	Schizophrenia simplex: mainly negative symptoms
F22	Delusional disorder: mainly delusions

In *paranoid* schizophrenia, delusions and hallucinations are most prominent, and catatonic and negative symptoms are less so. In *disorganized (hebephrenic)* schizophrenia, hallucinations and delusions are less likely but the patient suffers from formal thought and speech disorders and a lack of emotion. In *catatonic* schizophrenia, movement disturbances are most common, and these can range between the extremes of agitation and stupor (not reacting at all). It is characteristic that the patient has movement signs which sometimes result in specific positioning of the limbs.

If the patient suffers from *undifferentiated schizophrenia* or *schizophrenia simplex*, then none of these symptoms is prominent. However, negative symptoms are seen most frequently. If mainly delusions are prominent, a diagnosis of *delusional disorder* is made. This form is more common in patients aged over 50.

The doctor will know about all these different symptoms and can also use a structured assessment such as a scale of positive and negative syndromes.

7 THE MENTAL HEALTH CARE TEAM

The mental health care team is the team of people who collectively treat and look after patients with schizophrenia and other mental disorders. It ideally consists not only of the doctor but also of nurses, psychiatric social workers, psychologists and, more recently, case management professionals. All of these mental health care professionals should ideally work together constructively and inform the other members of the team about the current status of the patient. Whereas the doctor is mainly interested in specific illness-related questions such as the actual symptoms that the patient is experiencing, the other members of the team will have their own questions relating to their specific jobs. For example, the psychiatric social worker might ask about the living environment and if there are any specific problems in the workplace or home. The psychiatric nurse, depending on whether this is an in-patient or out-patient, works closely with the doctor preparing medications and dealing with illness-specific variables such as positive and negative symptoms. The case manager helps to coordinate the services and resources including the physical and social environment, including housing, psychiatric treatment, child health care, welfare entitlements, transportation, and family and social networks. It can be seen, therefore, that the mental health care team can provide a package of total care although it has to be said that all these facilities are unlikely to be available in all parts of the country.

8 HOW DOES SCHIZOPHRENIA PROGRESS AND WHAT ARE THE STAGES OF RECOVERY?

Schizophrenia is a long-term illness although it does have periods of remission when the symptoms are much less severe. This is shown diagrammatically in Figure 8.1. Here, the different phases of illness are shown as a graph. This starts below the level where symptoms can be noticed and then increases steadily as the first episode begins. It passes through the stage of mild symptoms and reaches a peak when the symptoms are severe. This is the first active phase of the illness. The symptoms then gradually disappear once the patient takes the proper medication (the recovery stage), and when they have gone completely

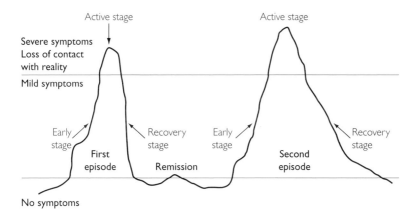

Figure 8.1 The different phases of illness in schizophrenia. The graph shows two episodes of symptoms separated by a period of remission when there are no symptoms. Each episode has an early phase, when symptoms begin, followed by an active phase when they are at their worst, and then a recovery stage during which they gradually disappear. (Modified from Nasrallah H, Smeltzer D. *Contemporary Diagnosis and Management of the Patient with Schizophrenia*, 2002, published by Handbooks in Health Care, Newtown, PA, USA)

19

the patient is in remission. Preventative medication (known as *prophylactic medication*, for example, antipsychotics or neuroleptics) together with proper psychosocial treatment from the rest of the mental health care team should then be given so that further episodes can be prevented. Unfortunately, subsequent episodes do become more difficult to treat and have a more drawn-out recovery stage. They also tend to come more quickly, that is, if untreated the next episode appears in a shorter time span than the previous one.

9 WHAT TREATMENTS ARE AVAILABLE?

Medical treatments

Drugs used in the treatment of schizophrenia are known as antipsychotic or neuroleptic drugs, and the first one, chlorpromazine, was developed in the 1950s. It is important to understand that none of these drugs can cure the disease but they are effective in reducing the symptoms. Having several different types of drugs available is very useful, since some of them are effective against different symptoms within the schizophrenic illness. This enables the doctor to be quite focused in the treatment given to any specific patient.

There are two groups of such drug: the newer atypical antipsychotics and the older neuroleptics. There are two significant differences between these two groups of drugs. The newer atypical antipsychotics show less specific side effects on some aspects of brain function (known as extrapyramidal side effects). They are also an effective treatment for all the symptoms of schizophrenia whereas the older drugs are mainly effective against the positive symptoms. The different types of medications are included in Table 9.1.

Table 9.1   Atypical antipsychotics and some older neuroleptics

Atypical antipsychotics	Older neuroleptics
Clozapine	Haloperidol*
Risperidone*	Fluphenazine*
Olanzapine	Zuclopenthixol*
Quetiapine	Levomepromazine
Zotepine	

*These drugs can also be given by injection and will last for a longer period (depot medication).

Based on the knowledge of a disturbance in the neurotransmitter dopamine and most likely also serotonin of patients with schizophrenia, there is a need to influence these neurotransmitter systems in order to treat the disease properly. Unfortunately, the medication affects not only the dopamine and serotonin systems but also other neurotransmitter systems like the *histaminergic* and the *cholinergic* neurons, resulting in side effects like weight gain and disturbance of cognition.

The older typical *neuroleptics* are quite effective for treatment of positive symptoms but unfortunately about half the patients on these drugs do experience unacceptable side effects, such as jerky movements or the inability to sit or stand still (extrapyramidal side effects). In order to overcome these side effects, another drug (biperiden) has to be given. However, although this drug can reduce the movement problems, it can cause other side effects like impaired cognition, dry mouth and constipation.

The atypical antipsychotics, of which *clozapine* was the first, have now changed the treatment of schizophrenia. Other new drugs of this type include *risperidone*, *olanzapine*, *quetiapine* and *zotepine*. These medications have the same antipsychotic potency as the older medications but substantially lower, or in some cases negligible, side effects. They are therefore superior to the older neuroleptic drugs in this respect. Of course, the real test is what patients think, and most report that with the newer type of medication they find it easier to concentrate and to think clearly, and also that they have either no or only mild acceptable side effects. Another common finding is that patients feel as they did before the disease started and that they participate more in social activities. The UK government body known as NICE (National Institute for Clinical Excellence) has recently endorsed the use of the atypical antipsychotics for use in all newly diagnosed patients and those existing patients who experienced unacceptable side effects with the older drugs.

Specifically, impaired cognition, the inability to think clearly, which is a core symptom of schizophrenia, is influenced positively by this group of medications, most likely through the influence of the serotonin 2 receptors which are blocked in cortical areas.

Since schizophrenia sometimes also results in agitation and hostility, it is worth mentioning that the newer drugs significantly improve these symptoms. However, if these drugs on their own or in combination with *neuroleptic drugs* are unable to control anxiety or agitation, then a benzodiazepine drug such as *lorazepam* can be added as a co-medication.

22

Table 9.2   Indications for long-term drug treatment in schizophrenia

Frequency of symptoms	Length of drug treatment before medication can be withdrawn
First manifestations	1–2 years antipsychotic treatment
2 to 3 episodes, or second episode within 1 year	2–5 years preventative treatment
Frequently recurring episodes with danger for the patient or for others	Fairly unlimited preventative treatment

Because schizophrenia is a long-term illness, there should be 1–2 years of antipsychotic treatment after the first manifestation of the condition. The basic treatment routine for the long-term is outlined in Table 9.2.

The treatment should last for 2–5 years if the patient suffers from a second or third manifestation or if there is a relapse within one year. Thereafter, together with the doctor and the mental health care team, a decision needs to be taken whether or not the medication should be taken for a longer period of time. Generally there should be no limit to the length of treatment if more than three manifestations have already been observed. In general, from the total population of patients with schizophrenia, 15% suffer from only one manifestation, 50% suffer from recurrent manifestations, and 35% suffer from a severe and also deteriorating course of the illness.

One of the most important aspects is the detection of signs of a relapse. This can often be achieved by the patient himself, or failing that, from the relatives. The main signs of relapse are listed in Table 9.3.

Table 9.3   Signs of relapse in schizophrenia

The most important issue for the prevention of relapse in schizophrenia is for the patient to take his or her medication as prescribed.

Signs of relapse
Lack of psychosocial engagement
Anxiety; restlessness; hostility
Depression; social isolation
'Strange' behaviour which does not belong to the personality
Suspiciousness; behaves as if he or she knows 'more'

The signs of relapse include a withdrawal from social situations, not taking medication, showing signs of anxiety and irritability, having sleep disturbances and changes in eating habits. If any of these symptoms appear, health care professionals should be approached rapidly.

With proper treatment, the symptoms of schizophrenia can, in most cases, be kept at bay. Hallucinations and delusions usually respond well to the antipsychotic drugs, and the other symptoms of schizophrenia (negative, affective and cognitive) can be treated effectively with the newer atypical antipsychotic drugs.

The treatment of schizophrenia includes drug as well as psychosocial treatment from members of the mental health care team. Since in most cases the treatment of schizophrenia is a long-term matter, the effectiveness of the medication should include its effect on positive, negative, cognitive and affective symptoms. In addition, the way in which the patient tolerates the taking of the medication, and how satisfied he or she is with the results, are of the utmost importance. Interestingly, patients judge the value of a medication on the tolerability whereas doctors in the past quite often looked at the effectiveness on target symptoms and could not value the tolerability very highly since there was no other medication available. This unfortunately led to the situation where patients did not take their medication.

Psychosocial treatments

Psychosocial treatments include individual psychotherapy, family therapy, group therapy, social skills training as well as case management. Most of these treatments are also used in other psychiatric disorders and have to be specifically tailored to the disease as well as to the individual patient. However, not all therapies used in other psychiatric diseases are also suitable for schizophrenia, and it is up to members of the mental health care team to assess each patient with regard to which therapy is best suited to their particular situation. Some, like insight-oriented psychodynamic psychotherapy, have been shown to be ineffective.

A few psychosocial approaches have been developed specifically for serious psychiatric disorders like schizophrenia. The primary goal of these interventions is to provide social support and an understanding of the illness and its management while emphasizing the importance of adherence to treatment, establishing a *rapport* and a therapeutic alliance with the patient, encouraging social functions, helping the patient to cope with the usual situations in life as well as focusing on the disability resulting from the disease in their daily activities.

This group of psychosocial and rehabilitative interventions include helping the patient function individually as well as within a family or small social circle. Cognitive or behavioural therapy has been developed to reduce the stress and interference with functioning due to psychotic symptoms. Residual symptoms can also be addressed with this approach.

Social skills training is a structured educational procedure that stresses the use of modelling, role playing and social reinforcement. Social interactions such as making a date or cashing a cheque are practised with the patient and entail specific verbal and non-verbal social skills. The inclusion of the family is always a very important step in the successful treatment of schizophrenia. Research has shown that expressed emotions, that is, those emotions expressed from the family towards the patient, whether positive or negative, need to be filtered out and kept from the patient. If this is not achieved, then some patients will experience a higher recurrence rate. Research has also shown that if the family are considered as part of the total treatment package, then the intervals between relapses become longer and the course of the disease is more favourable.

Supportive disease-specific psychotherapy, which includes psycho-education as well as strategies for management of the disease, should, of course, be given during all phases of the illness but most importantly in the subsequent phases.

10 COMMONLY ASKED QUESTIONS

Is schizophrenia a split personality?

This term is quite often used in everyday language but it is a misinterpretation of the meaning of the word, and gives the impression that people with schizophrenia behave as if they are two persons. There *is* a rare disease called *dissociative identity disorder* (previously known as *multi-personality disorder*) in which two or more distinct identities or personalities recurrently and alternately manifest themselves in a person's behaviour. Such patients report that each personality state can act rationally and generally remains in good contact with external reality. However, this condition is completely different from schizophrenia, and in schizophrenia no distinct identities are seen. The term 'split personality' refers to the fact that people with schizophrenia are *split off* from reality and when experiencing their symptoms, such as hallucinations and delusions, cannot always distinguish between what is real and what is not real.

Are people with schizophrenia dangerous to other people?

In general, patients who suffer from schizophrenia are no more dangerous than the general population. However, during the active phase of the illness there might be disease processes that make the sufferer feel that he or she is being persecuted or that voices tell the sufferer to do something. In such situations, it is possible that people with schizophrenia might have aggressions due to their illness. Later on, they may well question what was wrong with their actions. Difficult though it may be, it is important to understand the reasons for such behaviour, assuming of course that one is aware of the person's medical history.

I don't like taking tablets so I always try and take a few less than the doctor prescribed for me

Drug dosages for schizophrenia have been very carefully developed by researchers and drug companies. The doctor will always calculate the right amount based on the individual's particular condition and the state of his or her disease. Taking a lower dose in the mistaken belief that less medicine is a good thing is actually a very bad idea indeed. Not only may a lower dose be ineffective and not treat the symptoms but it could also increase the likelihood of a relapse. Patients should always take the dosage that has been prescribed by the doctor. Naturally, if they are experiencing side effects then this is a different issue, and they should go back to the doctor immediately to see if there are alternatives which are more tolerable.

Are the drugs used to treat schizophrenia addictive?

There is a general perception that the drugs used for the treatment of psychiatric disorders are addictive. For most of the drugs, this is not true. The antidepressants, antipsychotics and neuroleptics used in the treatment of schizophrenia are all non-addictive, as are the mood stabilizers which are used for the treatment of another psychiatric disorder called bipolar disorder. These are very safe drugs and they can be used without fear of their becoming addictive. There are, however, some drugs, like those of the benzodiazepine group such as *diazepam* which are used to treat anxiety, which do need to be taken with care in order that they do not become addictive. Doses of these drugs need to be monitored carefully by the doctor.

I've heard that antipsychotic drugs are very dangerous and I'm worried because my doctor has said that I should take them regularly

It is very important that you go and see your doctor and tell him or her that you are worried and exactly why you are worried. When taken as prescribed, antipsychotics are a well tolerated and effective medication. You may have heard that it is dangerous to take them in overdose but this is true for most drugs. This can be dangerous and you would probably need intensive care treatment. In most cases, your doctor will prescribe either one or two tablets of antipsychotics to be taken daily and you should stick exactly to this programme.

Would I be like a zombie if I take my drugs?

The new antipsychotic drugs have more or less replaced the older neuroleptics and therefore patients taking these medications do not experience the side effects, especially the movement-associated ones, of the older drugs. Some of the modern drugs, although by no means all of them, can have a sedative effect to start with, so there might be a feeling of sleepiness at the beginning of the treatment. However, this disappears after a few days of treatment. If the feeling of sleepiness or drowsiness continues, then the doctor or nurse should be told since they might advise you to change the amount of drugs you are taking or prescribe another medication.

11 CASE STUDIES

Case 1

A 24-year-old male patient with schizophrenia appeared in the emergency department of the local hospital, having been brought in by his mother. During the examination, he admitted that he heard voices telling him to move around in his little village. He was also sure that the doctor in his village, together with other people in the village, were against him. He said that over the last 4 weeks it had not been easy for him to fall asleep and even when he was asleep he was not sleeping soundly. He was not convinced that an in-patient treatment would be helpful. However, since he was sweaty and nervous he agreed that something was going wrong with his 'nerves' and he therefore agreed to stay in hospital for a short period. The patient was given two drugs: risperidone (one of the newer antipsychotic drugs), together with one of the benzodiazepine drugs for his anxiety. Although the patient initially felt a little sedated, he noticed that there was a lower level of anxiety in him and he found this to be a beneficial situation. He also trusted his medical care team to look after him properly. Gradually, the dose of the anti-anxiety drug could be reduced and eventually he was discharged with just one evening dose of the antipsychotic medication. His condition was diagnosed as *paranoid schizophrenia*.

Case 2

A 56-year-old man is working as a driver for a company and thinks that his wife has a lover. He is very jealous, and has some evidence that supports his suspicion. He views himself as a conservative person and his wife's infidelity is therefore unbearable for him and is something that he will not tolerate. His past medical history includes some alcohol abuse although not to a large extent. The wife consults the local general hospital and brings her husband in for an appointment. However, when he is in the hospital he realizes that everybody is against him and he gets very aggressive. Doctors give him an injection of a neuroleptic drug called haloperidol, which results in severe side effects affecting his movement. He is then transferred to the psychiatric unit and because of the side effects, his medication is changed to one of the newer drugs, known as an atypical antipsychotic. This drug is as effective as the older one but does not have the movement side effects when given in the correct dosage. The patient remains in hospital for 4 weeks during which time his treatment is stabilized, and after which he is discharged with instructions to take one dose every evening. After 6 months, this is reduced to a lower dose. Although he still has some suspicion about his wife, the drug treatment together with supportive psychotherapy is sufficient to allow him to carry on with life as normal. His condition was diagnosed as *delusional disorder.*

12   WEBSITES

The internet is being used increasingly by patients and their families who wish to learn more about their condition or problem. Although it is not a substitute for good health care, it can be a rich source of useful information if it is used properly.

There are several websites and self-help groups which may be useful and they are listed below. However, patients should talk to their doctors or other health care professionals about anything which they find on a website. Sadly, claims are sometimes made about treatments which are untrue. Medical treatments of any kind should never be ordered from a website without first discussing this with your doctor, nurse or pharmacist.

The following is just a very brief selection of websites relevant to schizophrenia. Many more can be found by writing *schizophrenia* in the search box of an internet search engine such as Google or Yahoo. The websites provide information which can be printed off and may also provide links to other organizations. They differ from the support groups listed in Chapter 13 since these are (mainly) charitable organizations that provide a personal and individual service whereby trained personnel will respond to specific queries from patients and/or family members.

- www.docguide.com
- www.mentalillness.com
- www.world-schizophrenia.org
- www.schizophrenia.mentalhelp.net
- www.psychiatry24x7.com
- www.schizophrenia.com
- www.rcpsych.ac.uk
- www.doh.gov.uk/mentalhealthcontact/orgs2.htm

Newsgroups and bulletin boards allow anyone with access to a computer and the internet to write a message or post a question to all the other people who use the newsgroup. Newsgroups can be useful if you want to ask a question or look for information, but one must be cautious. Users have no idea who has written the material or who is providing the advice, even if impressive sounding names and qualifications adorn the site. Often the people who reply are kind, sympathetic and understanding; sometimes, however, they can be also rude and unhelpful. Occasionally, people may recommend medication or other courses of action that they have personally found useful. However, it is possible that their recommendations might not have a scientific basis at all. So, be wary of what you read and do not necessarily accept everything as being true.

13   SUPPORT GROUPS

Support groups are usually charitable organizations whose aim is to provide practical and emotional support to sufferers and their families and carers. The most prominent groups in the United Kingdom are the following. Some of these have overseas branches but most other countries will also have their own local and national associations.

The National Schizophrenia Fellowship (now known as Rethink)

This organization is the largest charity in Europe that works with people who have severe mental illness. It operates more than 350 projects in the United Kingdom and more than 150 local support groups. They can be contacted directly for details of any projects in a chosen area. Contact details are:

RETHINK
30 Tabernacle Street
London EC2A 4DD
Head Office telephone: 020 7330 9100
National Advice Service: 020 8974 6814
Fax: 020 7330 9102
e-mail: info@nsf.org.uk
Website: www.nsf.org.uk

Schizophrenia Association of Great Britain

This organization provides help and advice to sufferers from schizo-phrenia and their families. Its additional aims are to raise awareness of the condition and to promote research into the causes. Contact details are:

Schizophrenia Association of Great Britain
Bryn Hyfryd
The Crescent
Bangor
Gwynedd LL57 2AG
Telephone and fax: 01248 354048
e-mail: info@sagb.co.uk
Website: www.sagb.co.uk

SANE

SANE is one of the major charities in the United Kingdom concerned with improving the lives of everyone affected by mental illness. It provides an extensive literature and sponsors research. Contact details are:

SANE
First floor
Cityside House
40 Adler Street
London E1 1EE
There are also offices in Bristol (0117 950 2140) and in Macclesfield (01625 429 050).
Telephone: 0845 767 8000
e-mail: london@sane.org.uk (at present, SANE cannot answer questions about mental illness by e-mail and such enquiries should be made by telephone)
Website: www.sane.org.uk

Mind

Mind is a leading mental health charity in the United Kingdom and works for a better life for those people who are diagnosed as mentally ill. Among its many activities, Mind publishes a wide variety of information fact sheets. Its telephone helpline is run by a team of trained information officers and volunteers. There is also an e-mail service. Contact details are:

Mind
15–19 Broadway
London E15 4BQ
There are also branches in Wales (029 2039 5123) and in
    Warwickshire (024 7641 4366).
Telephone: 08457 660 163
e-mail: contact@mind.org.uk
Website: www.mind.org.uk

Carers' National Association (CNA)

The CNA works to improve the recognition and services for carers by
drawing carers' issues to the attention of the Government and other
policy makers. It has a free telephone helpline for carers of elderly, ill,
or disabled relatives and friends. Contact details are:

Carers' National Association
20–25 Glasshouse Yard
London EC1A 4JT
Telephone: 020 7490 8818
Free helpline: 0808 808 7777
e-mail: internet@ukcarers.org
Website: www.carersuk.demon.co.uk

The Samaritans

The Samaritans is a charity that exists to provide confidential emotional
support to anyone who is despairing or suicidal. They provide a 24-
hour telephone service as well as an e-mail service which normally
responds within 24 hours. All the trained volunteers use the pseudo-
nym 'Jo'. Their parent organization, Befrienders International, has over
30 000 volunteer workers in 350 centres in 41 countries. Contact details
are:

Telephone: 08457 909090
e-mail: jo@befrienders.org
Websites: www.samaritans.org.uk; www.befrienders.org

INDEX

Note: page numbers in *italics* refer to figures and tables